TABLE OF CONTENTS

INTRODUCTION 3

FOODS TO EAT AND AVOID 7

CAUSES OF AUTOIMMUNE DISEASES 10

TREATMENT OF AUTOIMMUNE DISEASES 16

BENEFITS AUTOIMMUNE PALEO (AIP) DIET 23

BREAKFAST RECIPES FOR AUTOIMMUNE PALEO (AIP) DIET 29

LUNCH RECIPES FOR AUTOIMMUNE PALEO (AIP) DIET 42

DINNER RECIPES FOR AUTOIMMUNE PALEO (AIP) DIET 54

MAIN DISHES FOR AUTOIMMUNE PALEO (AIP) DIET . 66

CONCLUSION 79

INTRODUCTION

The Autoimmune Paleo Diet, often referred to as AIP, is a specialized version of the Paleo diet designed to help individuals with autoimmune conditions manage their symptoms and promote healing. Autoimmune diseases occur when the immune system mistakenly attacks healthy cells in the body, leading to inflammation and tissue damage. The AIP diet aims to reduce inflammation and support the immune system by eliminating specific foods that may trigger or exacerbate autoimmune responses.

Basic Principles:

Elimination of Trigger Foods:

The AIP diet involves the elimination of certain foods known to be common triggers for inflammation and autoimmune reactions.

These typically include grains, legumes, dairy, processed sugars, processed oils, eggs, nightshades (like tomatoes, peppers, and eggplants), nuts, and seeds.

Focus on Nutrient-Dense Foods:

The emphasis is on consuming nutrient-dense, whole foods. This includes a variety of vegetables, fruits, quality meats (grass-fed and pasture-raised), and fish.

Gut Health:

The diet recognizes the importance of gut health in autoimmune conditions. Foods that support gut healing, such as bone broth and fermented foods, are often included.

Anti-Inflammatory:

AIP is designed to be anti-inflammatory, aiming to reduce inflammation throughout the body. This is crucial in managing autoimmune conditions where chronic inflammation is a common feature.

Gradually reintroduce eliminated foods one at a time to identify specific triggers and gauge individual tolerance.

Individualization:

The AIP diet can be personalized based on individual responses and needs.

Consultation with Healthcare Professionals:

Before starting the AIP diet, especially if you have a diagnosed autoimmune condition, it's crucial to consult with healthcare professionals, such as a registered dietitian or a healthcare provider familiar with nutrition and autoimmune disorders. They can provide personalized guidance based on your health status and specific needs. Additionally, it's essential to monitor for nutrient deficiencies and make adjustments as needed.

Remember that the AIP diet is not a one-size-fits-all solution, and its effectiveness may vary from person to person. Always consult with healthcare professionals to create a comprehensive plan tailored to your unique health situation.

FOODS TO EAT AND AVOID

FOODS TO EAT

Vegetables:

A wide variety of colorful, non-nightshade vegetables are encouraged.

Fruits:

Berries and other fruits in moderation.

Meats:

High-quality, grass-fed or pasture-raised meats.

Fish:

Fatty fish rich in omega-3 fatty acids.

Healthy Fats:

Avocado, olive oil, coconut oil.

Bone Broth:

Supports gut health and provides essential nutrients.

Foods to Avoid

Grains:

Wheat, barley, rye, etc.

Legumes:

Beans, lentils, peanuts.

Dairy:

Milk, cheese, yogurt.

Processed Foods:

Anything with additives, preservatives, or artificial ingredients.

Processed Sugars:

Refined sugars and artificial sweeteners.

Nightshades:

Tomatoes, peppers, eggplants, and certain spices.

Nuts and Seeds:

Due to their potential to cause inflammation and irritation.

Implementation:

Elimination Phase:

Start with a strict elimination phase where you remove all potential trigger foods for a set period (commonly 30 days).

CAUSES OF AUTOIMMUNE DISEASES

Autoimmune diseases occur when the immune system, which is designed to protect the body from harmful invaders like bacteria and viruses, mistakenly attacks healthy cells. The exact causes of autoimmune diseases are not fully understood, and they likely involve a combination of genetic, environmental, and hormonal factors. Here are some key factors associated with the development of autoimmune diseases:

Genetic Factors:

There is often a genetic predisposition to autoimmune diseases. Certain genes may make individuals more susceptible to developing these conditions. However, having a genetic predisposition does not guarantee that a person will develop an autoimmune disease.

Environmental Triggers:

Various environmental factors may contribute to the development or exacerbation of autoimmune diseases. These can include infections, exposure to certain chemicals, and other environmental toxins. In some cases, an infection may trigger an autoimmune response as the immune system reacts to both the infectious agent and the body's own cells.

Hormonal Factors:

Autoimmune diseases are more prevalent in women than in men, suggesting a hormonal influence. Changes in hormone levels, such as those that occur during puberty, pregnancy, and menopause, can impact the immune system and contribute to the development of autoimmune conditions.

Leaky Gut Syndrome:

Some theories propose that a condition known as "leaky gut" may contribute to autoimmune diseases. Leaky gut occurs when the intestinal lining becomes more permeable, allowing substances that should be confined to the digestive tract to enter the bloodstream. This can trigger an immune response.

Stress:

Chronic stress has been implicated in the development and exacerbation of autoimmune diseases. Stress hormones can influence the immune system, potentially contributing to an autoimmune response.

Dietary Factors:

While the role of diet in autoimmune diseases is complex and varies between individuals, some dietary factors may influence the immune system. For example, certain proteins in gluten and dairy products have been suggested to contribute to autoimmune reactions in susceptible individuals.

Epigenetic Changes:

Epigenetic modifications, which involve changes in gene expression without altering the underlying DNA sequence, may play a role in the development of autoimmune diseases. Environmental factors can influence epigenetic changes.

Microbiome Dysbiosis:

The balance of microorganisms in the gut (microbiome) is increasingly recognized as playing a role in immune system regulation. Imbalances in the microbiome (dysbiosis) have been associated with autoimmune diseases.

It's important to note that autoimmune diseases are a diverse group of conditions, and different diseases may have different underlying causes and risk factors. Additionally, the interplay between genetic susceptibility and environmental triggers is complex and not fully understood. Research in this field is ongoing, and our understanding of autoimmune diseases continues to evolve. If you suspect you have an autoimmune condition or have been diagnosed with one, it is crucial to work closely with healthcare professionals to manage symptoms and develop an appropriate treatment plan.

TREATMENT OF AUTOIMMUNE DISEASES

The treatment of autoimmune diseases typically involves managing symptoms, suppressing excessive immune responses, and, in some cases, modifying the course of the disease. It's important to note that there is no cure for most autoimmune diseases, and treatment often focuses on improving quality of life and preventing complications. The specific approach to treatment can vary depending on the type of autoimmune disease, its severity, and individual factors. Here are common strategies used in the treatment of autoimmune diseases:

Medications:

Immunosuppressive Drugs: These drugs work to suppress the immune system and reduce inflammation. Examples include corticosteroids, disease-modifying antirheumatic drugs (DMARDs), and biologics. The choice of medication depends on the specific autoimmune disease and its severity.

Nonsteroidal Anti-Inflammatory Drugs (NSAIDs): These drugs help control pain and inflammation in conditions such as rheumatoid arthritis and lupus.

Pain Medications: In some cases, pain management medications may be prescribed to alleviate discomfort.

Hormone Replacement Therapy: For autoimmune diseases influenced by hormonal factors, hormone replacement therapy may be considered.

Dietary and Lifestyle Modifications:

Anti-Inflammatory Diet: Some individuals with autoimmune diseases find relief from symptoms by adopting an anti-inflammatory diet. This may include the elimination of certain trigger foods and the incorporation of foods that support overall health.

Regular Exercise: Physical activity can help improve joint function, reduce inflammation, and enhance overall well-being. Exercise programs should be tailored to individual capabilities and limitations.

Stress Management: Chronic stress can exacerbate autoimmune symptoms. Stress management techniques such as meditation, yoga, and relaxation exercises may be beneficial.

Adequate Sleep: Quality sleep is essential for overall health and may play a role in managing autoimmune conditions.

Physical and Occupational Therapy:

Physical therapists can provide exercises and techniques to improve joint function and mobility.

Occupational therapists may help individuals manage daily activities and adapt to limitations caused by the autoimmune disease.

Surgery:

In some cases, surgery may be necessary to address complications of autoimmune diseases. For example, joint replacement surgery for individuals with severe rheumatoid arthritis or gastrointestinal surgery for certain inflammatory bowel diseases.

Management of Specific Symptoms:

Symptomatic relief measures may include medications or interventions targeted at specific symptoms, such as pain, fatigue, or skin issues.

Monitoring and Follow-up:

Regular monitoring of symptoms, disease activity, and potential side effects of medications is essential. Adjustments to treatment plans may be made based on individual responses and disease progression.

Patient Education:

Understanding the nature of the autoimmune disease, treatment options, and self-management strategies is crucial. Patient education helps individuals actively participate in their care and make informed decisions.

It's important to emphasize that the management of autoimmune diseases is often a collaborative effort between the individual and a healthcare team, which may include rheumatologists, immunologists, primary care physicians, physical therapists, and other specialists depending on the specific condition. Treatment plans are typically tailored to the individual, considering factors such as age, overall health, and the specific features of the autoimmune disease.

If you or someone you know is dealing with an autoimmune disease, it's recommended to consult with healthcare professionals for personalized advice and a comprehensive treatment plan.

BENEFITS AUTOIMMUNE PALEO (AIP) DIET

The Autoimmune Paleo (AIP) Diet is designed to help manage autoimmune conditions by reducing inflammation and supporting overall health. While individual responses to the diet may vary, here are some potential benefits associated with following the AIP Diet:

1. Reduced Inflammation:

The AIP Diet emphasizes nutrient-dense, anti-inflammatory foods, which may help in reducing systemic inflammation, a common feature of autoimmune diseases.

2. Identifying Trigger Foods:

Through the elimination and reintroduction phases, individuals can identify specific foods that may trigger autoimmune responses, allowing for a more personalized approach to managing their condition.

3. Gut Health Improvement:

The inclusion of gut-healing foods like bone broth and fermented foods may contribute to improved gut health. This is significant, as the health of the gut is linked to the overall function of the immune system.

4. Nutrient-Dense Diet:

The focus on whole, nutrient-dense foods provides essential vitamins, minerals, and antioxidants, supporting overall health and potentially addressing nutrient deficiencies common in autoimmune conditions.

5. Symptom Management:

Many individuals report improvements in symptoms such as joint pain, fatigue, skin issues, and digestive problems when following the AIP Diet.

6. Weight Management:

The AIP Diet's emphasis on whole foods and the elimination of processed foods may support healthy weight management.

7. Improved Energy Levels:

Some individuals report increased energy levels and reduced fatigue, which can be significant for those dealing with chronic autoimmune conditions.

8. Enhanced Quality of Life:

Managing autoimmune diseases can be challenging, and the AIP Diet may contribute to an improved quality of life by addressing **symptoms and promoting overall well-being.**

9. Complementary to Medical Treatment:

The AIP Diet is often used as a complementary approach alongside medical treatment. It's important to note that the diet should be undertaken with guidance from healthcare professionals.

10. Mind-Body Connection:

The emphasis on stress management, adequate sleep, and overall well-being recognizes the interconnectedness of the mind and body, potentially contributing to a holistic approach to health.

11. Potential for Long-Term Lifestyle Changes:

Some individuals find that the AIP Diet serves as a foundation for long-term lifestyle changes, encouraging ongoing mindful eating **habits and overall health consciousness.**

12. Community Support:

Engaging with the AIP community can provide support, encouragement, and shared experiences. Online forums, social media groups, and resources offer a sense of community for individuals navigating the challenges of autoimmune conditions and dietary changes.

13. Personal Empowerment:

The AIP Diet encourages individuals to take an active role in managing their health. Understanding how different foods affect their well-being empowers individuals to make informed choices about their diet and lifestyle.

Important Consideration:

It's crucial to approach the AIP Diet with caution and under the guidance of healthcare professionals, especially if you have a diagnosed autoimmune condition. Additionally, individual responses to the diet can vary, and what works for one person may not work for another. It's recommended to work closely with healthcare providers, including registered dietitians or nutritionists familiar with autoimmune conditions, to create a personalized and sustainable plan that meets your specific needs.

BREAKFAST RECIPES FOR AUTOIMMUNE PALEO (AIP) DIET

Certainly! Here are some Autoimmune Paleo (AIP) diet-friendly recipes with ingredients and instructions:

1. ROASTED SWEET POTATO AND CARROT SOUP:

Ingredients:

2 medium sweet potatoes, peeled and diced

3 large carrots, peeled and sliced

1 onion, chopped

2 cloves garlic, minced

4 cups bone broth

1 teaspoon ground turmeric

Salt and pepper to taste

2 tablespoons coconut oil

Instructions:

Preheat oven to 400°F (200°C).

Toss sweet potatoes, carrots, onion, and garlic with coconut oil.

Roast in the oven for 30-40 minutes or until vegetables are tender.

Transfer roasted vegetables to a pot, add bone broth, turmeric, salt, and pepper.

Simmer for 15-20 minutes.

Blend the soup until smooth using an immersion blender.

Adjust seasoning and serve.

2. BAKED LEMON HERB CHICKEN:

Ingredients:

4 boneless, skinless chicken breasts

1 lemon, juiced

2 tablespoons fresh parsley, chopped

1 tablespoon fresh rosemary, chopped

1 tablespoon fresh thyme, chopped

2 cloves garlic, minced

Salt and pepper to taste

2 tablespoons olive oil

Instructions:

Preheat oven to 375°F (190°C).

In a bowl, combine lemon juice, parsley, rosemary, thyme, garlic, salt, and pepper.

Place chicken breasts in a baking dish and pour the lemon herb mixture over them.

Drizzle with olive oil.

Bake for 25-30 minutes or until chicken is cooked through.

3. ZUCCHINI NOODLES WITH PESTO:

Ingredients:

4 medium zucchinis, spiralized

1 cup fresh basil leaves

1/2 cup fresh parsley leaves

1/4 cup pine nuts

1/4 cup extra-virgin olive oil

1 clove garlic, minced

Salt and pepper to taste

Optional: nutritional yeast (AIP-friendly)

Instructions:

In a food processor, combine basil, parsley, pine nuts, olive oil, garlic, salt, and pepper.

Process until smooth to make the pesto.

Toss spiralized zucchini with the pesto.

Optional: sprinkle with nutritional yeast for a cheesy flavor.

4. SALMON AND AVOCADO SALAD:

Ingredients:

2 salmon fillets, grilled or baked

2 avocados, diced

1 cucumber, sliced

2 cups mixed greens

2 tablespoons olive oil

1 tablespoon lemon juice

Salt and pepper to taste

Instructions:

Flake the cooked salmon into bite-sized pieces.

In a bowl, combine salmon, avocado, cucumber, and mixed greens.

In a separate bowl, whisk together olive oil, lemon juice, salt, and pepper.

Drizzle the dressing over the salad and toss gently.

5. GARLIC AND HERB ROASTED BRUSSELS SPROUTS:

Ingredients:

1 pound Brussels sprouts, halved

3 tablespoons olive oil

2 cloves garlic, minced

1 teaspoon dried thyme

1 teaspoon dried rosemary

Salt and pepper to taste

Instructions:

Preheat oven to 400°F (200°C).

Toss Brussels sprouts with olive oil, garlic, thyme, rosemary, salt, and pepper.

Spread them on a baking sheet.

Roast for 20-25 minutes or until crispy on the edges.

6. AIP-FRIENDLY GUACAMOLE:

Ingredients:

3 avocados, mashed

1 lime, juiced

1/4 cup red onion, finely chopped

1/4 cup fresh cilantro, chopped

1 clove garlic, minced

Salt to taste

Instructions:

In a bowl, combine mashed avocados, lime juice, red onion, cilantro, and garlic.

Mix well and add salt to taste.

Serve with vegetable sticks or AIP-friendly crackers.

7. HERB-ROASTED TURKEY BREAST:

Ingredients:

1 bone-in, skin-on turkey breast

2 tablespoons fresh sage, chopped

2 tablespoons fresh thyme, chopped

2 tablespoons fresh rosemary, chopped

3 tablespoons olive oil

Salt and pepper to taste

Instructions:

Preheat oven to 325°F (165°C).

In a bowl, combine sage, thyme, rosemary, olive oil, salt, and pepper.

Rub the herb mixture over the turkey breast.

Roast for approximately 2-2.5 hours or until the internal temperature reaches 165°F (74°C).

8. AIP-FRIENDLY CAULIFLOWER RICE:

Ingredients:

1 head cauliflower, grated or processed into rice-sized pieces

2 tablespoons coconut oil

1 teaspoon turmeric

Salt and pepper to taste

Fresh parsley for garnish

Instructions:

In a skillet, heat coconut oil over medium heat.

Add cauliflower rice and turmeric.

Sauté for 5-7 minutes or until cauliflower is tender.

Season with salt and pepper.

Garnish with fresh parsley before serving.

9. TURMERIC GINGER CARROT SOUP:

Ingredients:

1 pound carrots, peeled and chopped

1 onion, chopped

2 cloves garlic, minced

1 tablespoon fresh ginger, grated

1 teaspoon ground turmeric

4 cups bone broth

2 tablespoons coconut oil

Salt and pepper to taste

Instructions:

In a pot, sauté onions, garlic, and ginger in coconut oil until fragrant.

Add carrots, turmeric, bone broth, salt, and pepper.

Bring to a boil, then reduce heat and simmer until carrots are tender.

Blend the soup until smooth using an immersion blender.

Adjust seasoning and serve.

10. AIP-FRIENDLY BERRY SMOOTHIE:

Ingredients:

1 cup mixed berries (e.g., blueberries, strawberries)

1 banana

1 cup coconut milk

1 tablespoon collagen powder (optional)

Ice cubes

Instructions:

In a blender, combine berries, banana, coconut milk, and collagen powder.

Blend until smooth.

Add ice cubes and blend again until desired consistency is reached.

LUNCH RECIPES FOR AUTOIMMUNE PALEO (AIP) DIET

11. LEMON HERB BAKED COD:

Ingredients:

4 cod fillets

2 tablespoons fresh parsley, chopped

1 tablespoon fresh thyme, chopped

1 lemon, sliced

2 tablespoons olive oil

Salt and pepper to taste

Instructions:

Preheat oven to 375°F (190°C).

Place cod fillets in a baking dish.

Drizzle with olive oil and sprinkle with parsley, thyme, salt, and pepper.

Top with lemon slices.

Bake for 15-20 minutes or until fish flakes easily.

12. AIP CHICKEN AND VEGETABLE STIR-FRY:

Ingredients:

2 chicken breasts, thinly sliced

2 cups broccoli florets

1 bell pepper, sliced

1 zucchini, sliced

2 tablespoons coconut aminos

1 tablespoon fresh ginger, grated

2 tablespoons coconut oil

Salt to taste

Instructions:

In a skillet, heat coconut oil over medium heat.

Add chicken and cook until browned.

Add broccoli, bell pepper, and zucchini.

Stir in coconut aminos, ginger, and salt.

Cook until vegetables are tender.

13. AIP BEEF AND SWEET POTATO STEW:

Ingredients:

1 pound beef stew meat

2 sweet potatoes, peeled and diced

1 onion, chopped

2 cloves garlic, minced

4 cups beef broth

1 teaspoon dried oregano

1 teaspoon dried thyme

Salt and pepper to taste

2 tablespoons coconut oil

Instructions:

In a pot, heat coconut oil over medium heat.

Brown beef stew meat.

Add onions and garlic, sauté until softened.

Add sweet potatoes, beef broth, oregano, thyme, salt, and pepper.

Simmer for 1-2 hours or until beef is tender.

14. AIP BROCCOLI AND BACON SALAD:

Ingredients:

4 cups broccoli florets

6 slices AIP-compliant bacon, cooked and crumbled

1/4 cup red onion, finely chopped

1/4 cup AIP-friendly mayonnaise

1 tablespoon apple cider vinegar

Salt and pepper to taste

Instructions:

Blanch broccoli in boiling water for 2 minutes, then plunge into ice water.

In a bowl, combine broccoli, bacon, and red onion.

In a small bowl, whisk together mayonnaise, apple cider vinegar, salt, and pepper.

Pour the dressing over the salad and toss to coat.

15. AIP SHRIMP AND AVOCADO SALAD:

Ingredients:

1 pound shrimp, peeled and deveined

2 avocados, diced

1 cucumber, sliced

1/4 cup fresh cilantro, chopped

2 tablespoons olive oil

1 tablespoon lime juice

Salt and pepper to taste

Instructions:

In a skillet, heat olive oil over medium heat.

Cook shrimp until pink and opaque.

In a bowl, combine shrimp, avocados, cucumber, and cilantro.

In a small bowl, whisk together lime juice, salt, and pepper.

Drizzle the dressing over the salad and toss gently.

16. AIP TURMERIC CHICKEN SOUP:

Ingredients:

2 chicken breasts, shredded

4 cups chicken broth

2 carrots, peeled and sliced

2 celery stalks, sliced

1 onion, chopped

2 cloves garlic, minced

1 teaspoon ground turmeric

2 tablespoons coconut oil

Salt and pepper to taste

Instructions:

In a pot, sauté onions and garlic in coconut oil until softened.

Add shredded chicken, carrots, celery, chicken broth, turmeric, salt, and pepper.

Simmer for 20-25 minutes or until vegetables are tender.

17. AIP CAULIFLOWER AND LEEK MASH:

Ingredients:

1 head cauliflower, chopped

2 leeks, chopped

2 tablespoons coconut oil

1/4 cup coconut milk

Salt and pepper to taste

Instructions:

Steam cauliflower and leeks until tender.

In a blender, combine steamed cauliflower, leeks, coconut oil, coconut milk, salt, and pepper.

Blend until smooth.

18. AIP BAKED CINNAMON APPLES:

Ingredients:

4 apples, cored and sliced

1 tablespoon coconut oil

1 teaspoon ground cinnamon

1/4 cup coconut cream

Instructions:

Preheat oven to 375°F (190°C).

In a baking dish, toss apple slices with coconut oil and cinnamon.

Bake for 20-25 minutes or until apples are tender.

Drizzle with coconut cream before serving.

19. AIP LEMON ROSEMARY ROASTED CHICKEN THIGHS:

Ingredients:

8 chicken thighs, bone-in, skin-on

1 lemon, juiced

2 tablespoons fresh rosemary, chopped

2 cloves garlic, minced

2 tablespoons olive oil

Salt and pepper to taste

Instructions:

Preheat oven to 400°F (200°C).

In a bowl, combine lemon juice, rosemary, garlic, olive oil, salt, and pepper.

Place chicken thighs in a baking dish and coat with the lemon rosemary mixture.

Bake for 30-35 minutes or until chicken is cooked through.

20. AIP BERRY COCONUT PANNA COTTA:

Ingredients:

2 cups mixed berries (e.g., blueberries, raspberries)

1 can (14 ounces) coconut milk

2 tablespoons maple syrup (optional)

1 tablespoon gelatin

Instructions:

In a saucepan, heat coconut milk and maple syrup over low heat.

Sprinkle gelatin over the mixture and whisk until dissolved.

Remove from heat and let it cool.

In serving glasses, alternate layers of mixed berries and coconut mixture.

Refrigerate for at least 4 hours or until set.

DINNER RECIPES FOR AUTOIMMUNE PALEO (AIP) DIET

21. AIP BEEF AND BROCCOLI STIR-FRY:

Ingredients:

1 pound grass-fed beef, thinly sliced

3 cups broccoli florets

1 onion, thinly sliced

2 cloves garlic, minced

2 tablespoons coconut aminos

1 tablespoon fresh ginger, grated

2 tablespoons coconut oil

Salt to taste

Instructions:

In a skillet, heat coconut oil over medium heat.

Add sliced beef and cook until browned.

Add broccoli, onion, garlic, coconut aminos, ginger, and salt.

Stir-fry until the broccoli is tender and the beef is cooked.

22. AIP CREAMY ASPARAGUS SOUP:

Ingredients:

1 pound asparagus, trimmed and chopped

1 onion, chopped

2 cloves garlic, minced

4 cups bone broth

1/2 cup coconut cream

2 tablespoons coconut oil

Salt and pepper to taste

Instructions:

In a pot, sauté onions and garlic in coconut oil until softened.

Add asparagus and bone broth. Simmer until asparagus is tender.

Blend the soup until smooth.

Stir in coconut cream and season with salt and pepper.

23. AIP SPAGHETTI SqUASH WITH BOLOGNESE SAUCE:

Ingredients:

1 spaghetti squash, halved and seeds removed

1 pound ground beef

1 onion, chopped

2 cloves garlic, minced

1 can (14 ounces) crushed tomatoes (AIP-compliant)

2 tablespoons fresh basil, chopped

2 tablespoons coconut oil

Salt and pepper to taste

Instructions:

Preheat oven to 375°F (190°C).

Roast spaghetti squash halves in the oven until fork-tender.

In a skillet, sauté onions and garlic in coconut oil until softened.

Add ground beef and cook until browned.

Stir in crushed tomatoes, basil, salt, and pepper.

Scoop the spaghetti squash into strands and top with the bolognese sauce.

24. AIP CILANTRO LIME CHICKEN SKEWERS:

Ingredients:

1 pound chicken thighs, cut into cubes

1/4 cup fresh cilantro, chopped

2 tablespoons olive oil

2 tablespoons lime juice

1 teaspoon ground cumin (optional, omit for strict AIP)

Salt and pepper to taste

Instructions:

In a bowl, combine chicken cubes, cilantro, olive oil, lime juice, cumin (if using), salt, and pepper.

Thread the chicken onto skewers.

Grill or bake until cooked through.

25. AIP LEMON GARLIC ROASTED BRUSSELS SPROUTS:

Ingredients:

1 pound Brussels sprouts, halved

2 tablespoons olive oil

2 cloves garlic, minced

1 lemon, juiced

Salt and pepper to taste

Instructions:

Preheat oven to 400°F (200°C).

Toss Brussels sprouts with olive oil, garlic, lemon juice, salt, and pepper.

Spread them on a baking sheet.

Roast for 20-25 minutes or until crispy on the edges.

26. AIP THAI-INSPIRED COCONUT CHICKEN SOUP:

Ingredients:

1 pound chicken breast, thinly sliced

4 cups chicken broth

1 can (14 ounces) coconut milk

1 zucchini, spiralized

2 tablespoons fresh cilantro, chopped

2 tablespoons lime juice

1 tablespoon fish sauce (optional, omit for strict AIP)

Salt to taste

Instructions:

In a pot, bring chicken broth to a simmer.

Add sliced chicken, coconut milk, zucchini, cilantro, lime juice, fish sauce (if using), and salt.

Simmer until chicken is cooked through and flavors meld.

27. AIP CHOCOLATE AVOCADO PUDDING:

Ingredients:

2 ripe avocados

1/4 cup coconut milk

3 tablespoons carob powder

2 tablespoons maple syrup

1 teaspoon vanilla extract (AIP-compliant)

Pinch of salt

Instructions:

In a blender, combine avocados, coconut milk, carob powder, maple syrup, vanilla extract, and a pinch of salt.

Blend until smooth and creamy.

Chill in the refrigerator before serving.

28. AIP TUNA SALAD LETTUCE WRAPS:

Ingredients:

2 cans (5 ounces each) tuna, drained

1/4 cup AIP-friendly mayonnaise

1 tablespoon fresh dill, chopped

1 tablespoon capers, chopped

Lettuce leaves for wrapping

Instructions:

In a bowl, combine tuna, mayonnaise, dill, and capers.

Mix well.

Spoon the tuna salad into lettuce leaves and wrap.

29. AIP ROSEMARY ROASTED ROOT VEGETABLES:

Ingredients:

2 sweet potatoes, peeled and diced

2 parsnips, peeled and diced

2 carrots, peeled and diced

2 tablespoons coconut oil

1 tablespoon fresh rosemary, chopped

Salt and pepper to taste

Instructions:

Preheat oven to 400°F (200°C).

Toss sweet potatoes, parsnips, and carrots with coconut oil, rosemary, salt, and pepper.

Spread them on a baking sheet.

Roast for 30-40 minutes or until vegetables are tender.

30. AIP BLUEBERRY COCONUT POPSICLES:

Ingredients:

2 cups blueberries

1 can (14 ounces) coconut milk

2 tablespoons honey (optional, omit for strict AIP)

1 teaspoon vanilla extract (AIP-compliant)

Instructions:

In a blender, combine blueberries, coconut milk, honey (if using), and vanilla extract.

Blend until smooth.

Pour the mixture into popsicle molds.

Freeze until solid.

MAIN DISHES FOR AUTOIMMUNE PALEO (AIP) DIET

31. AIP CABBAGE AND BEEF SKILLET:

Ingredients:

1 pound ground beef

1 head green cabbage, shredded

1 onion, chopped

2 cloves garlic, minced

2 tablespoons coconut oil

1 teaspoon dried oregano

Salt and pepper to taste

Instructions:

In a skillet, heat coconut oil over medium heat.

Add ground beef and cook until browned.

Add onions and garlic, sauté until softened.

Stir in shredded cabbage, oregano, salt, and pepper.

Cook until cabbage is tender.

32. AIP TURMERIC-GINGER SALMON:

INGREDIENTS:

4 salmon fillets

1 tablespoon fresh turmeric, grated

1 tablespoon fresh ginger, grated

2 tablespoons olive oil

1 lemon, sliced

Salt and pepper to taste

Instructions:

Preheat oven to 375°F (190°C).

In a bowl, mix turmeric, ginger, olive oil, salt, and pepper.

Place salmon fillets on a baking sheet.

Coat each fillet with the turmeric-ginger mixture.

Top with lemon slices.

Bake for 15-20 minutes or until salmon is cooked through.

33. AIP SWEET POTATO BREAKFAST HASH:

Ingredients:

2 sweet potatoes, peeled and diced

1 pound ground turkey

1 onion, chopped

2 tablespoons coconut oil

1 teaspoon dried thyme

Salt and pepper to taste

Fresh parsley for garnish

Instructions:

In a skillet, heat coconut oil over medium heat.

Add ground turkey and cook until browned.

Add onions and sweet potatoes, sauté until sweet potatoes are tender.

Season with thyme, salt, and pepper.

Garnish with fresh parsley before serving.

34. AIP LEMON HERB GRILLED CHICKEN:

Ingredients:

4 chicken breasts

1 lemon, juiced

2 tablespoons fresh basil, chopped

2 tablespoons fresh mint, chopped

2 tablespoons olive oil

Salt and pepper to taste

Instructions:

In a bowl, combine lemon juice, basil, mint, olive oil, salt, and pepper.

Marinate chicken breasts in the mixture for at least 30 minutes.

Grill until chicken is cooked through.

35. AIP BUTTERNUT SqUASH SOUP:

Ingredients:

1 butternut squash, peeled and diced

1 onion, chopped

2 cloves garlic, minced

4 cups bone broth

1 teaspoon ground cinnamon

2 tablespoons coconut oil

Salt and pepper to taste

Instructions:

In a pot, sauté onions and garlic in coconut oil until softened.

Add butternut squash and bone broth.

Simmer until squash is tender.

Blend the soup until smooth.

Season with cinnamon, salt, and pepper.

36. AIP CHICKEN LIVER PÂTÉ:

Ingredients:

1/2 pound chicken livers

1/2 cup coconut oil, melted

1 onion, chopped

2 cloves garlic, minced

1 teaspoon dried thyme

Salt and pepper to taste

Instructions:

In a skillet, sauté onions and garlic in coconut oil until softened.

Add chicken livers and cook until no longer pink in the center.

Transfer the mixture to a food processor.

Blend until smooth.

Season with thyme, salt, and pepper.

Refrigerate before serving.

37. AIP PLANTAIN PANCAKES:

Ingredients:

2 ripe plantains

2 tablespoons coconut flour

2 tablespoons coconut oil

1/2 teaspoon baking soda

Pinch of salt

AIP-friendly cooking fat for greasing

Instructions:

In a blender, combine plantains, coconut flour, coconut oil, baking soda, and salt.

Blend until smooth.

Heat a skillet over medium heat and grease with AIP-friendly cooking fat.

Pour small amounts of batter onto the skillet to form pancakes.

Cook until bubbles form, then flip and cook the other side.

38. AIP CUCUMBER AVOCADO SALAD:

Ingredients:

2 cucumbers, sliced

2 avocados, diced

1/4 cup fresh dill, chopped

2 tablespoons olive oil

1 tablespoon apple cider vinegar

Salt and pepper to taste

Instructions:

In a bowl, combine cucumbers, avocados, and dill.

In a small bowl, whisk together olive oil, apple cider vinegar, salt, and pepper.

Pour the dressing over the salad and toss gently.

39. AIP PUMPKIN SOUP:

Ingredients:

2 cups pumpkin puree

1 onion, chopped

2 cloves garlic, minced

4 cups bone broth

1/2 teaspoon ground ginger

1/2 teaspoon ground cinnamon

2 tablespoons coconut oil

Salt and pepper to taste

Instructions:

In a pot, sauté onions and garlic in coconut oil until softened.

Add pumpkin puree and bone broth.

Simmer until the soup is heated through.

Season with ginger, cinnamon, salt, and pepper.

40. AIP MANGO-COCONUT CHICKEN SKEWERS:

Ingredients:

1 pound chicken thighs, cut into cubes

1 mango, peeled and diced

1/4 cup coconut milk

2 tablespoons fresh cilantro, chopped

1 tablespoon lime juice

Salt and pepper to taste

Instructions:

In a bowl, combine chicken cubes, diced mango, coconut milk, cilantro, lime juice, salt, and pepper.

Thread the chicken onto skewers.

Grill or bake until chicken is cooked through.

NOTE: Remember to adjust recipes based on your individual tolerances and preferences, and consult with a healthcare professional or a registered dietitian for personalized advice.

Enjoy these AIP-friendly recipes as part of a balanced and nourishing diet.

CONCLUSION

In conclusion, the Autoimmune Paleo (AIP) diet is a therapeutic approach aimed at managing autoimmune conditions by reducing inflammation and supporting overall health. It involves the elimination of potential trigger foods and focuses on nutrient-dense, anti-inflammatory options. The AIP diet places emphasis on whole foods, such as vegetables, fruits, lean proteins, and healthy fats, while avoiding grains, dairy, legumes, nuts, and seeds.

The potential benefits of the AIP diet include reduced inflammation, identification of trigger foods through an elimination and reintroduction process, improved gut health, and symptom management for individuals with autoimmune conditions. Additionally, the AIP diet may contribute to a nutrient-dense and well-balanced eating pattern, supporting overall health and well-being.

It's important to note that the AIP diet should be approached with caution and under the guidance of healthcare professionals, especially for individuals with diagnosed autoimmune conditions. Each person's response to the diet can vary, and it's crucial to ensure that nutritional needs are met.

Moreover, the AIP diet goes beyond dietary changes and often includes lifestyle modifications, such as stress management, adequate sleep, and physical activity. This holistic approach recognizes the interconnectedness of factors influencing health and aims to address them collectively.

As with any dietary regimen, individual preferences, tolerances, and responses should be taken into account. Consulting with a healthcare professional or a registered dietitian who is knowledgeable about autoimmune conditions is advisable to create a personalized and sustainable plan tailored to an individual's specific health needs. The AIP diet can be a valuable tool for some individuals in managing autoimmune conditions, but it is not a one-size-fits-all solution, and its effectiveness may vary from person to person.

www.ingramcontent.com/pod-product-compliance
Lightning Source LLC
Chambersburg PA
CBHW050745260726
48661CB00001B/415